# EMPOWERED PATH TO PREGNANCY:

## FROM ONE FELLOW PCOS WARRIOR TO ANOTHER

### VOLUME 1: PCOS ROADMAP

BY: KELLY TAYLOR

## TABLE OF CONTENTS

Hello my fellow PCOS Warrior! Thank you so much for purchasing my *Empowered Path to Pregnancy: From One Fellow PCOS Warrior To Another* - **Volume 1: PCOS ROADMAP.** I'm thrilled to be a part of your journey! Just a bit of business before we dive in:

## DISCLAIMERS

I am not a medical professional, and this guide is not intended to replace professional medical advice, diagnosis, or treatment. The information shared here is based on my personal experiences and research to provide guidance and support. Always consult a qualified healthcare provider before making any changes to your health, lifestyle, or treatment plan. Your healthcare provider can offer advice tailored specifically to your individual needs and circumstances.

Book Design by Kelly Taylor

# STEP 1: UNDERSTANDING PCOS

## WHAT IS PCOS?

Polycystic Ovary Syndrome (PCOS) is a complex hormonal disorder that affects 1 in 10 women of reproductive age. Despite the name, PCOS isn't just about ovaries or cysts; it's a multifaceted condition involving an imbalance of reproductive and metabolic hormones. This imbalance can lead to a range of symptoms that affect not only the reproductive system but also a woman's overall health and quality of life.

## HOW PCOS AFFECTS OVULATION & FERTILITY

*1. Hormonal Imbalance*

At its core, PCOS involves an imbalance of hormones. Women with PCOS typically produce higher-than-normal levels of androgens, also known as "male hormones," such as testosterone. This excess of androgens can interfere with ovulation—the process of releasing an egg from the ovary each month. For many women, the elevated androgen levels lead to irregular or absent menstrual cycles, making it harder to conceive.

*2. Insulin Resistance and Metabolic Issues*

Another critical factor in PCOS is insulin resistance, which means the body's cells don't respond as well to insulin, a hormone that helps regulate blood sugar levels. As a result, the body produces more insulin to compensate. This can increase androgen production even further, exacerbating PCOS symptoms. Insulin resistance also raises the risk of developing Type 2 diabetes, cardiovascular disease, and weight gain, especially around the abdomen.

### *3. The Formation of Ovarian Cysts*

Despite the term "polycystic," not every woman with PCOS will develop ovarian cysts, and having ovarian cysts alone doesn't mean someone has PCOS. For those who do, the "cysts" in PCOS are actually immature follicles that haven't released an egg. Instead of completing ovulation, these follicles accumulate in the ovaries, appearing like "cysts" on an ultrasound. This accumulation can contribute to irregular menstrual cycles and may lead to ovulation problems.

## COMMON SYMPTOMS, CAUSES & DIAGNOSIS OF PCOS

### *1. Symptoms*

The symptoms of PCOS can vary widely, and not every woman will experience the same combination. Some of the most common include:

- **Irregular Periods:** Women with PCOS often have fewer than eight menstrual cycles a year, or none at all. This irregularity is typically one of the first signs of the condition.

- **Excess Hair Growth (Hirsutism):** Due to high androgen levels, many women with PCOS experience excess hair growth on areas like the face, chest, stomach, and back. This can be distressing and is often one of the more visible symptoms.
- **Acne and Oily Skin:** Androgens can cause skin problems, leading to persistent acne on the face, back, and chest, often beyond teenage years.
- **Weight Gain or Difficulty Losing Weight:** Because of insulin resistance, many women with PCOS find it challenging to manage their weight, especially around the abdomen, regardless of diet or exercise.
- **Thinning Hair on the Scalp:** While body hair may increase, scalp hair can thin, leading to hair loss or pattern baldness similar to male hair loss.
- **Mood Disorders:** Women with PCOS are at a higher risk for depression and

anxiety, partly due to the physical symptoms and hormonal imbalance.

- **Darkening of the Skin**: Some women may develop dark patches of skin, particularly around the neck, armpits, or under the breasts (a condition called acanthosis nigricans), often associated with insulin resistance.

### *2. Causes*

The exact cause of PCOS remains unknown, though it's believed to result from a combination of genetic & environmental factors. It tends to run in families, indicating a genetic component, and factors like lifestyle, stress, and diet can exacerbate symptoms.

### *3. Diagnosis*

There is no single test to diagnose PCOS, so doctors rely on a combination of medical history, physical exams, blood tests, and ultrasounds. Most practitioners use the Rotterdam Criteria, which require at least two of the following for a diagnosis:

- Irregular or absent menstrual cycles
- High levels of androgens (either through blood tests or physical symptoms)
- Polycystic ovaries on ultrasound

# STEP 2: PREPARING FOR PREGNANCY WITH PCOS

## BUILDING YOUR SUPPORT TEAM

When preparing for pregnancy with PCOS, one of the most important steps is to build a strong, supportive team around you. PCOS is a complex condition, and having a reliable support system can make all the difference in managing the challenges it presents. This team can help you navigate the emotional, physical, and medical aspects of preparing for pregnancy, and empower you to take charge of your health and fertility.

***1. Your Healthcare Providers: The Core of Your Team***

Your first step in building a support team is to find a healthcare provider who understands PCOS and is supportive of your goals. Whether it's a gynecologist, endocrinologist, or a fertility specialist, it's crucial to work with a provider who listens to your concerns, offers evidence-based treatments, and supports your choice to pursue natural conception.

For women with PCOS, treatment can be varied depending on the symptoms and individual needs. A fertility specialist can help if conception is proving difficult, while an endocrinologist can assist in managing hormonal imbalances.

Alternatively, a gynecologist familiar with PCOS may provide general care. Regular checkups, blood work, and ultrasounds to monitor hormone levels and ovarian health are essential for maintaining fertility health.

**Key Questions to Ask Your Healthcare Provider:**

- What natural methods can I use to regulate my hormones and cycles?
- How can I improve my fertility with PCOS?

- What supplements or lifestyle changes do you recommend?
- How can we monitor my progress toward pregnancy?

***2. Holistic Practitioners: Supporting Your Body and Mind***

PCOS affects not just the body but also the mind, leading to stress, anxiety, and sometimes, depression. Holistic practitioners can play a key role in helping you heal your body naturally and manage the emotional stress that often comes with the condition.

Consider adding an acupuncturist, nutritionist, or naturopathic doctor to your team. Acupuncture has been shown to help regulate menstrual cycles, reduce stress, and improve ovarian function in women with PCOS. A nutritionist specializing in hormone health can assist you in creating a balanced, PCOS-friendly diet that supports fertility and overall wellness. Naturopaths can provide natural remedies like herbal supplements or lifestyle advice that work alongside conventional medical treatments.

**Holistic Approaches to Consider:**

- Acupuncture to regulate hormones and improve circulation to the ovaries
- Nutritional counseling to balance blood sugar and reduce inflammation
- Stress reduction techniques such as yoga or mindfulness practices

### *3. Emotional Support: Friends, Family, and Partner*

The emotional impact of PCOS can be significant. It's essential to build a support system that includes friends, family, and your partner who can offer encouragement, understanding, and a listening ear. Your loved ones are your emotional foundation during this journey, and their support can ease the mental and emotional load.

Having a partner who is fully engaged in the process can be especially empowering. Pregnancy preparation is a team effort, and it's important to communicate openly about feelings, challenges, and hopes. Your partner can help by attending doctor's appointments, managing stress together, and providing emotional support through the ups and downs.

**Building Emotional Support:**

- Share your journey with trusted friends and family who will offer encouragement.
- Seek out a support group, either in person or online, to connect with others who understand the unique struggles of PCOS and pregnancy preparation.
- Involve your partner by keeping them informed and engaged in the process.

### *4. Mental Health Professionals: Navigating Stress and Anxiety*

Preparing for pregnancy with PCOS can bring about stress, anxiety, and feelings of isolation. Seeing a counselor or therapist who specializes in reproductive health or infertility can provide a safe space to express your emotions. Cognitive-behavioral therapy (CBT) has been shown to help women manage stress and negative thought patterns during the fertility journey.

A mental health professional can help you develop coping strategies, manage the pressure of trying to conceive, and improve your overall mental well-being. They can also help you process feelings of grief, disappointment, or frustration that may arise during this process.

**Mental Health Support Options:**

- Therapy to manage anxiety, stress, and depression related to PCOS and infertility
- Stress reduction techniques, including mindfulness and relaxation exercises
- Group therapy or support groups for women facing similar challenges

***5. Your Own Determination: The Key to Success***

While your healthcare providers, holistic practitioners, and support system are all vital parts of your team, the most important member is YOU! Your commitment, determination, and self-care practices are essential to successfully preparing for pregnancy with PCOS.

Take the time to educate yourself about PCOS, fertility, and natural conception methods. Be proactive in managing your health, making lifestyle changes, and advocating for your needs. Your mental, emotional, and physical well-being are crucial, and by taking ownership of your journey, you'll empower yourself to take the necessary steps toward healing and conception.

**Empowering Yourself:**

- Educate yourself about PCOS and fertility
- Set realistic goals and be patient with your progress
- Practice self-care and prioritize your mental and emotional health

Building a strong support team is one of the most important steps in preparing for pregnancy with PCOS. By surrounding yourself with knowledgeable healthcare providers, holistic practitioners, emotional support from loved ones, and mental health professionals, you'll be better equipped to navigate the challenges of PCOS and embrace your fertility journey with confidence. With the right team, you'll feel empowered to take control of your health, heal holistically, and work toward the dream of becoming a mother.

## TRACKING YOUR CYCLE & OVULATION

Tracking your menstrual cycle is one of the most empowering tools when trying to conceive with PCOS. Many women with PCOS experience irregular cycles, which can make it harder to predict ovulation and pinpoint the most fertile days. However, by tracking key indicators, you can gain insight into your body's rhythms, identify patterns, and increase your chances of conception. Here's how you can track your cycle effectively and some tools that can help:

### *1. Use a Fertility Tracker App*

Fertility tracker apps are a convenient way to monitor your cycle, record symptoms, and predict ovulation. These apps use data inputs such as your period start and end dates, cycle length, and other symptoms to calculate your fertile window. These apps can:

- Predict ovulation based on past cycle data.
- Help you track symptoms like bloating, mood swings, and cramps that could correlate with ovulation.
- Give insights into your most fertile days, based on your cycle's length and past patterns.

### *2. Monitor Ovulation Using Basal Body Temperature (BBT)*

Basal body temperature (BBT) is your body's temperature at rest, typically taken first thing in the morning before you get out of bed. Tracking your BBT daily can help you pinpoint ovulation because your temperature rises slightly after ovulation due to increased progesterone levels.

**How to Track BBT:**

- Use a digital basal thermometer, which is more sensitive than a regular thermometer. It reads temperature to the nearest tenth of a degree.
- Take your temperature at the same time each morning, ideally before getting up or moving around.
- Record your temperature in a chart or an app (many fertility tracker apps also allow you to track your BBT).

***3. Observe Changes in Cervical Mucus***

Your cervical mucus (CM) changes throughout your menstrual cycle, and tracking these changes can help identify your most fertile days. In the days leading up to ovulation, your cervical mucus becomes clear, stretchy, and slippery, resembling raw egg whites. This type of mucus helps sperm travel to the egg, making it the ideal time to try to conceive.

**How to Track Cervical Mucus:**

- Check your cervical mucus daily, ideally after using the bathroom but before wiping.
- Track the changes in consistency, color, and texture:

**Post-period:** Dry or sticky mucus
**Pre-ovulation:** Creamy, lotion-like mucus
**Ovulation:** Clear, slippery, egg white-like mucus.

Some women use cervical mucus charts to track these changes, and many fertility apps allow you to record this symptom.

***4. Use Urinary Ovulation Predictor Kits (OPKs)/Ovulation Test Kits***

Urinary ovulation predictor kits (OPKs), also known as LH surge tests, are one of the most popular and convenient methods for tracking ovulation. These over-the-counter tests detect the luteinizing hormone (LH) surge in your urine, which occurs 12-36 hours before ovulation. This surge signals that ovulation is near, making it the ideal time for conception.

**How Urinary Ovulation Predictor Kits (OPKs) Work:**

- **Use the Test Daily:** Start testing a few days before your expected ovulation based on your cycle length. If you have irregular cycles due to PCOS, you may need to start testing earlier in your cycle.
- **Test at the Same Time Each Day**: For consistent results, it's important to test at the same time each day, ideally in the afternoon, as LH levels can fluctuate throughout the day.
- **Interpret the Results:** Most LH test kits, such as Clearblue or First Response, will show a test line and a control line. If the test line is as dark or darker than the control line, it indicates a positive result, meaning ovulation is about to occur.
- **Track Over Several Days:** For women with PCOS, it can take a few days of testing to detect the surge due to

hormonal imbalances. Keeping track of the results can help you pinpoint when ovulation is most likely to happen.

*If you get a positive result on your ovulation test kit, aim to have intercourse within the next 12-36 hours to maximize conception chances, as this aligns with peak fertility.*

For women with PCOS, ovulation may not happen on a predictable schedule, but using an OPK in combination with BBT tracking can help you catch the LH surge and confirm that ovulation is imminent. It's also helpful to track this with your BBT or cervical mucus observations for a more comprehensive picture of your fertility.

**Pros of Urinary Ovulation Predictor Kits (OPKs):**

- **Accuracy:** When used correctly, these kits are highly accurate in detecting the LH surge and predicting ovulation.

- **Convenience**: Easy to use at home, and results are available within minutes.
- **Affordable:** Many brands offer cost-effective options for regular use, especially if you're not tracking every day.

With PCOS, there is often hormonal fluctuations, and you may not ovulate every cycle so ovulation tests might show a "false positive" or detect multiple LH surges. However, combining these tests with other methods like BBT and cervical mucus tracking can help you better understand your ovulation patterns.

By using urinary ovulation predictor kits (OPKs) along with other tracking methods, you'll have an even more powerful
toolkit for identifying the optimal time for conception, helping you increase your chances of pregnancy with PCOS.

### *5. Keep Track of Menstrual Cycle Length and Regularity*

Tracking your period's start and end dates, as well as its length, is important for women with PCOS. While your cycles may be irregular, consistently noting your cycle length and any changes (such as longer or shorter cycles) can help you understand your body's pattern. Regularly tracking these aspects can also help identify when your cycles become more regular, signaling potential improvements in hormone balance.

*If you have longer cycles, say 35-45 days, you may not ovulate every month. By tracking your cycle length and understanding your body's pattern, you can start to predict when your cycle might be more predictable and identify fertile windows.*

While PCOS can make conceiving a challenge, tracking your menstrual cycle, ovulation, and cervical mucus can empower you to take control of your fertility journey.

By using fertility apps, monitoring BBT, observing changes in cervical mucus, and incorporating ovulation predictor kits, you can improve your chances of conception and feel more confident about your fertility. These tools help you understand your body's patterns, identify your fertile window, and take the necessary steps toward pregnancy, even with PCOS.

# STEP 3: DIETARY & LIFESTYLE MODIFICATIONS

Boosting fertility with PCOS often involves lifestyle changes that support hormone balance, improve insulin sensitivity, and enhance reproductive health. Here are some key areas to focus on:

## NUTRITIONAL TIPS FOR PCOS

***1. Adopt a Balanced, PCOS-Friendly Diet:*** Focus on whole grains, lean proteins, healthy fats, and fiber-rich fruits and vegetables. These foods help regulate blood sugar and reduce inflammation, both crucial for managing PCOS. High-fiber foods, like vegetables, beans, and whole grains, can slow sugar absorption, which helps stabilize insulin levels. Healthy fats from sources like olive oil, avocados, and nuts support hormone production and overall health.

*2.Incorporate Anti-Inflammatory Foods:*
Chronic inflammation is common in PCOS and can worsen symptoms. Foods rich in omega-3 fatty acids, such as fatty fish (salmon, mackerel), chia seeds, flaxseeds, and walnuts, can help reduce inflammation and support hormone regulation. Turmeric, ginger, and dark leafy greens are also known for their anti-inflammatory properties, which can promote a healthier environment for reproductive health.

*3. Focus on Low-Glycemic and High-Fiber Foods:*
A low-glycemic diet emphasizes foods that cause minimal blood sugar fluctuations, essential for managing insulin resistance in PCOS. Low-glycemic foods include legumes, leafy greens, whole grains, and berries, which help maintain stable blood sugar levels and prevent insulin spikes. Fiber also aids in gut health, supporting the microbiome, which plays a role in hormone balance.

## IMPORTANCE OF WEIGHT MANAGEMENT

***1. Maintain a Healthy Weight:***

For women with PCOS, weight management can significantly impact symptoms and fertility. Excess weight, especially abdominal fat, can increase insulin resistance and inflammation. Achieving and maintaining a healthy weight can improve insulin sensitivity, support regular menstrual cycles, and balance hormone levels. Studies show that even a modest weight loss of 5-10% can help restore ovulation and improve the likelihood of conception.

***2. Exercise Regularly:***

A mix of cardiovascular exercise (like walking, swimming, or cycling) and strength training (such as weightlifting, resistance bands, or yoga) can help manage weight, improve metabolism, and regulate hormones. Cardiovascular exercise aids in burning calories and managing weight, while strength training increases lean muscle, enhancing metabolism and insulin sensitivity, which are essential for PCOS management.

***3. Reduce Inflammation:***

For women with PCOS, managing inflammation can help improve symptoms and overall health. Extra body fat, particularly visceral fat, can produce inflammatory markers that exacerbate inflammation. Engaging in regular physical activity helps lower these markers, supporting both metabolic and reproductive health.

***4. Minimize Toxins & Environmental Chemicals:***

**Reduce Exposure to Endocrine Disruptors:** Certain chemicals found in plastics, pesticides, and personal care products can disrupt hormone function, potentially impacting fertility. Choosing natural, non-toxic products whenever possible, along with avoiding plastic containers that may contain BPA or phthalates, can support hormone health and reduce your exposure to harmful chemicals. Look for glass containers, stainless steel options, or BPA-free plastics to reduce exposure.

**Quit Smoking:** Smoking can significantly reduce fertility by affecting hormone levels and decreasing blood flow to the ovaries. Quitting smoking not only enhances general health but can also improve your chances of conceiving naturally. Smoking cessation has been shown to positively impact hormone balance and overall reproductive health.

**Limit Alcohol Consumption:** While moderate alcohol intake may not significantly affect fertility, excessive alcohol use can disrupt hormone balance and may reduce fertility. Limiting or avoiding alcohol while trying to conceive may help improve hormone stability and support a healthier environment for conception.

## EXERCISE & ITS IMPACT ON FERTILITY

***1. Improve Insulin Sensitivity:***

Insulin resistance is a common issue in PCOS, contributing to irregular cycles, weight gain, and challenges with ovulation. Regular exercise, particularly a combination of aerobic and strength-training workouts, improves how the body uses insulin, promoting more stable blood sugar levels. Improved insulin sensitivity can positively impact hormone levels, enhancing ovulation and, consequently, fertility.

***2. Regulate Hormones and Enhance Circulation:***

PCOS often causes hormonal imbalances, including elevated androgen levels, which can interfere with ovulation. Exercise helps regulate these hormones by lowering androgen levels and increasing estrogen levels, promoting more regular cycles. Additionally, exercise increases blood flow, improving circulation to reproductive organs. Enhanced circulation aids in delivering essential nutrients, supporting a healthier ovarian and uterine environment for conception.

***3. Reduce Stress:***

Dealing with PCOS can be stressful, especially when managing symptoms and fertility challenges. Exercise releases endorphins, the body's natural mood boosters, which help reduce stress and improve overall well-being. It also lowers cortisol levels, the stress hormone, which can impact hormone balance. Reduced stress levels contribute to better sleep, improved mental health, and more stable hormones, positively impacting fertility.

However, it's important to consult with a healthcare provider before starting any new exercise program, as individual needs may vary. A balanced approach to exercise, along with a healthy diet and lifestyle choices, can be a powerful tool in your fertility journey.

# STEP 4: FERTILITY TESTING FOR YOU & YOUR SPOUSE

When trying to conceive, fertility testing plays a critical role in identifying potential obstacles to pregnancy and determining the best course of action. For both women with PCOS and their partners, comprehensive fertility testing helps pinpoint any underlying issues that may be hindering conception. Below is an expanded overview of common fertility tests for both partners that are essential in the pursuit of a successful pregnancy.

## FERTILITY TESTING FOR WOMEN

For women, fertility testing typically includes evaluating ovulation, hormone levels, ovarian reserve, and reproductive health. These tests help to determine whether conditions like PCOS, endometriosis, or blocked fallopian tubes are interfering with conception.

*1. Hormone Level Testing*

- **Follicle Stimulating Hormone (FSH) Test:** FSH is involved in egg development and ovulation. High levels of FSH can indicate poor ovarian reserve, which may be a concern for women trying to conceive.
- **Luteinizing Hormone (LH) Test:** LH works closely with FSH to regulate ovulation. Testing LH levels can help determine ovulation timing and detect abnormalities.
- **Estradiol Test:** This hormone helps regulate the menstrual cycle and is essential for ovulation. It can also help assess the health of the ovaries and the endometrial lining.
- **Progesterone Test:** This test is typically done 7 days after ovulation to confirm whether the body is producing enough progesterone to support a potential pregnancy.

- **Thyroid Function Tests:** Thyroid imbalances (hypothyroidism or hyperthyroidism) can interfere with fertility and menstrual regularity, so testing for thyroid hormones (TSH, Free T4, and Free T3) is essential.
- **Prolactin Test:** Prolactin is a hormone that supports lactation. Elevated prolactin levels can interfere with ovulation and fertility.
- **Anti-Müllerian Hormone (AMH) Test:** This blood test measures the levels of AMH, a hormone produced by the ovaries that indicates the number of eggs a woman has left. It provides insight into ovarian reserve, especially important for women with PCOS.

### *2. Pelvic Ultrasound*

A pelvic ultrasound is a non-invasive imaging test that can provide valuable information about the health of the ovaries, uterus, and fallopian tubes. It can detect: ovarian cysts or follicles (a common issue in PCOS), usterine fibroids, polyps, or structural abnormalities that could affect implantation, endometriosis or scar tissue that might block the fallopian tubes or affect the uterus.

*3. Hysterosalpingography (HSG)*

This is an X-ray procedure used to assess the health of the uterus and fallopian tubes. A dye is injected into the uterus, and X-rays are taken to confirm if the fallopian tubes are open and if the uterine cavity is normal. Blocked tubes or uterine abnormalities can be significant barriers to conception.

*4. Laparoscopy*

This minimally invasive surgical procedure is often performed if a woman has been struggling with infertility for an extended period or if there is suspicion of endometriosis, pelvic adhesions, or other conditions that may not be visible through other tests. A camera is inserted into the abdomen to evaluate the pelvic organs directly.

### *5. Ovarian Reserve Testing*

For women with PCOS, ovarian reserve testing helps determine how many eggs are available for fertilization. In addition to the AMH test, this might include:

- **Antral Follicle Count (AFC):** An ultrasound measurement of small follicles within the ovaries that could potentially develop into eggs.
- **Day 3 FSH and Estradiol:** These hormone tests, when done on day 3 of the menstrual cycle, help assess ovarian reserve and function.

## FERTILITY TESTING FOR MEN

Fertility testing for men is also essential, as male factors contribute to about one-third of infertility cases. The following tests are commonly recommended for evaluating male fertility.

### *1. Semen Analysis*

Semen analysis is the primary test for assessing male fertility. It examines the following key factors:

- **Sperm count:** The number of sperm in a semen sample. A low sperm count can reduce the chances of conception.
- **Sperm motility:** The ability of sperm to swim effectively toward the egg. Poor motility can decrease fertility.
- **Sperm morphology:** The shape and size of sperm. Abnormal sperm morphology can impact the ability of sperm to fertilize an egg.
- **Semen volume and viscosity:** This test measures how much semen is ejaculated and its consistency, which can affect sperm movement and the chances of successful fertilization.

*2. Hormone Testing*

- **Testosterone levels:** Testosterone is crucial for sperm production. Low levels can indicate underlying issues like hypogonadism, which can affect fertility.
- **FSH and LH levels:** These hormones regulate sperm production. Low levels may indicate a problem with the pituitary gland or testes.

- **Prolactin levels:** Elevated prolactin can inhibit testosterone production and sperm development, leading to infertility.

*3. Genetic Testing*

In some cases, genetic testing may be recommended if there are concerns about male fertility. This may include:

- **Karyotyping:** To check for chromosomal abnormalities that could affect sperm production or fertility.
- **Y-chromosome microdeletion testing:** This tests for specific genetic issues related to sperm production that could affect male fertility.

*4. Scrotal Ultrasound*

This imaging test can detect abnormalities in the testes, such as varicoceles (enlarged veins), which can cause infertility by increasing testicular temperature and reducing sperm production.

*5. Post-Ejaculation Urinalysis*

This test checks for retrograde ejaculation, a condition where sperm flows backward into the bladder rather than being expelled. This could affect sperm count in semen samples.

*6. Testicular Biopsy*

If semen analysis indicates an absence of sperm (azoospermia), a testicular biopsy may be performed to determine if sperm is being produced in the testes but is not making its way into the semen.

## TESTING FOR BOTH PARTNERS: COMPREHENSIVE EVALUATION

Fertility is a partnership and testing both partners together ensures a thorough understanding of potential issues on both sides. A fertility specialist may suggest additional testing based on the results from each partner's initial assessments. The following tests may be considered for both partners:

***1. Infectious Disease Screening***

Certain sexually transmitted infections (STIs) or other infections can affect fertility. Screening for diseases like chlamydia, gonorrhea, and HIV can be an important part of fertility testing.

***2. Genetic Carrier Screening***

Genetic carrier screening tests both partners for inherited genetic disorders, like cystic fibrosis, sickle cell anemia, or Tay-Sachs disease, that could potentially be passed to the child. This can help assess the risk of passing on genetic conditions to offspring.

***3. Fertility and Lifestyle Assessments***

A discussion about lifestyle factors that impact fertility is essential. Both partners should be evaluated for:

- **Diet and nutrition** (impact on egg and sperm health)
- **Exercise habits** (excessive exercise or lack of it can affect fertility)
- **Substance use** (alcohol, smoking, drugs, and caffeine can reduce fertility)

- **Stress management** (high stress levels can interfere with hormonal balance and conception).

Fertility testing is an essential step for both partners when trying to conceive. For women with PCOS, tests like hormone assessments, ovarian reserve testing, and ultrasound can help identify factors affecting fertility, while men's fertility testing primarily focuses on sperm quality, count, and motility. A comprehensive evaluation of both partners ensures that no underlying issues are overlooked and allows fertility specialists to recommend personalized treatment plans, improving the chances of a successful pregnancy. By addressing both male and female fertility factors early on, couples can take proactive steps toward achieving their dreams of becoming parents.

# STEP 5: MEDICAL TREATMENTS

## MEDICAL TREATMENTS

Medications to aid ovulation are seen as a key component of treatment for women with PCOS who are struggling with infertility. Since PCOS often leads to irregular or absent ovulation due to hormonal imbalances, these medications are designed to stimulate the ovaries to produce eggs, making conception more likely. Below is an expanded look at the different types of medications used to aid ovulation in women with PCOS:

***1. Clomiphene Citrate (Clomid):***

Clomiphene citrate is one of the most commonly prescribed medications for inducing ovulation in women with PCOS. It is an oral medication that works by stimulating the pituitary gland to release more follicle stimulating hormone (FSH), which in turn encourages the ovaries to produce eggs.

- **How it works:** Clomid blocks estrogen receptors in the hypothalamus, tricking the brain into thinking estrogen levels are low. This stimulates the release of FSH and luteinizing hormone (LH), which prompts the ovaries to start ovulating.
- **Success rates:** Clomid has a success rate of about 60-80% for stimulating ovulation in women with PCOS. However, ovulation does not always lead to pregnancy, and multiple cycles may be required.
- **Side effects:** Common side effects include hot flashes, mood swings, bloating, and headaches. In some cases, Clomid can also lead to ovarian cysts, which can cause pain or discomfort.
- **Considerations:** It's usually the first-line treatment and is typically prescribed for a few cycles. If Clomid

does not work after several cycles, other medications may be considered.

*2. Letrozole (Femara)*

Letrozole is another oral medication used to stimulate ovulation, particularly in women with PCOS. It was originally developed as a treatment for breast cancer but has shown promise in inducing ovulation in women who have difficulty conceiving.

- **How it works:** Letrozole is an aromatase inhibitor, which means it reduces estrogen production by blocking the enzyme responsible for converting androgens into estrogen. The decrease in estrogen signals the brain to release FSH, stimulating ovulation.
- **Success rates:** Letrozole has been found to be more effective than Clomid in some studies, particularly in women with PCOS who do not respond to Clomid. It has a higher ovulation rate and is associated with a lower risk of multiples (e.g. twins).

- **Side effects:** Side effects are generally mild and may include fatigue, dizziness, headaches, and hot flashes. Unlike Clomid, Letrozole has a lower risk of causing ovarian cysts.
- **Considerations:** Letrozole is typically prescribed as the first-line treatment if Clomid fails or if a woman prefers an alternative with a better ovulation rate and fewer side effects.

*3. Gonadotropins (FSH and LH injections)*
Gonadotropins are injectable hormones used when oral medications like Clomid or Letrozole are unsuccessful in stimulating ovulation. These injections contain FSH and LH (follicle-stimulating hormone and luteinizing hormone), which directly stimulate the ovaries to produce eggs.

- **How it works:** Gonadotropins are injected directly into the bloodstream and help stimulate the ovaries to produce mature eggs. This treatment is more controlled than Clomid or Letrozole, as the dosage of hormones can be adjusted to optimize the chances of ovulation.

- **Success rates:** Gonadotropins are highly effective, with success rates for ovulation ranging from 60-90%. However, they come with a higher risk of multiple pregnancies (e.g., twins or triplets).
- **Side effects:** Potential side effects include ovarian hyperstimulation syndrome (OHSS), a condition where the ovaries become swollen and painful. Other risks include multiple pregnancies and ovarian cysts.
- **Considerations:** Gonadotropins are often used in combination with ovulation monitoring (e.g., ultrasounds and blood tests) to track follicle development and optimize the timing of ovulation. This treatment is typically considered when other medications haven't been successful.

***4. Metformin (Glucophage)***

Metformin is an oral medication primarily used to treat type 2 diabetes, but it is also prescribed to women with PCOS to improve insulin sensitivity and help regulate ovulation. While it does not directly stimulate ovulation, it can be an important part of treatment for those with insulin resistance, which is common in women with PCOS.

- **How it works:** Metformin works by improving the body's sensitivity to insulin, reducing insulin resistance. Lower insulin levels can help reduce androgen production, which can improve ovulation and menstrual regularity in women with PCOS.
- **Success rates:** Metformin has been shown to improve ovulation in women with PCOS who also have insulin resistance, particularly when combined with other ovulation-stimulating medications like Clomid.
- **Side effects:** Common side effects include gastrointestinal issues such as nausea, diarrhea, and abdominal discomfort, especially when first starting metformin. These side effects

often lessen over time as the body adjusts to the medication.

- **Considerations:** Metformin is often used in combination with other medications, such as Clomid or Letrozole, to help improve fertility outcomes. It is particularly helpful for women who have difficulty ovulating due to insulin resistance.

***5. Bromocriptine***

Bromocriptine is used in women with PCOS who have high levels of prolactin, a hormone produced by the pituitary gland. Elevated prolactin levels can interfere with ovulation and fertility. Bromocriptine works by lowering prolactin levels and restoring normal ovulatory cycles.

- **How it works:** Bromocriptine is a dopamine agonist that inhibits the production of prolactin, which can improve ovulation in women with PCOS who have elevated prolactin levels.
- **Success rates:** It is effective for women with prolactin imbalances and may be

used when other medications have not worked.

- **Side effects:** Potential side effects include dizziness, nausea, and headaches. These are usually temporary and resolve once the body adjusts to the medication.

# STEP 6: NATURAL SUPPLEMENTS & HERBAL REMEDIES

## NATURAL SUPPLEMENTS FOR PCOS

### *1. Inositol Supplements*

Inositol, particularly myo-inositol and D-chiro inositol, are supplements often used in the treatment of PCOS. These compounds are thought to help improve insulin sensitivity, regulate menstrual cycles, and promote ovulation.

- **Purpose:** Inositol is a natural compound that helps improve insulin sensitivity, lower androgen levels, and promote regular menstrual cycles.
- **How it Works:** Myo-inositol and D-chiro inositol, specifically, are commonly used for PCOS. They mimic insulin's effects in the body and

help regulate menstrual cycles and ovulation.

- **Dosage:** A common dose is 2,000 mg of myo-inositol and 50 mg of D-chiro inositol daily, but it's always best to follow product guidelines or consult a healthcare provider.

*2. Omega-3 Fatty Acids (Fish Oil)*

- **Purpose:** Omega-3s help reduce inflammation, support heart health, and improve insulin sensitivity.
- **How it Works:** By decreasing inflammation, omega-3s can help reduce PCOS symptoms like acne and may lower testosterone levels, which can improve symptoms like hirsutism (excess hair growth).
- **Dosage:** Typical doses range from 1,000 to 3,000 mg daily.

*3. Vitamin D*

- **Purpose:** Vitamin D supports immune function, insulin sensitivity, and hormonal balance.

- **How it Works:** Many women with PCOS are deficient in vitamin D. Correcting this deficiency can improve menstrual regularity, fertility, and mood.
- **Dosage:** Depending on blood levels, doses of 1,000–5,000 IU per day may be recommended, but blood tests can help determine the right amount.

*4. Magnesium*

- **Purpose:** Magnesium helps regulate blood sugar, supports relaxation, and improves mood.
- **How it Works:** Magnesium reduces insulin resistance and helps manage stress, which can have a positive impact on PCOS symptoms like menstrual irregularity and anxiety.
- **Dosage:** A typical dose is 300–400 mg daily, often taken in the form of magnesium citrate or magnesium glycinate for better absorption.

*5. Zinc*

- **Purpose:** Zinc has anti-inflammatory properties, reduces acne, and may help reduce androgen levels.
- **How it Works:** Zinc helps with hormone regulation and may reduce symptoms like hirsutism, acne, and hair loss. It also supports immune health and wound healing.
- **Dosage:** 10-30 mg per day is a common dose.

*6. N-Acetyl Cysteine (NAC)*

- **Purpose:** NAC supports liver detoxification, reduces inflammation, and improves insulin sensitivity.
- **How it Works:** NAC helps boost levels of glutathione, a powerful antioxidant, which helps improve insulin resistance and may support fertility in women with PCOS.
- **Dosage:** Commonly, 600–1,200 mg per day is recommended.

*7. Chromium*

- **Purpose:** Chromium supports insulin function and blood sugar regulation.
- **How it Works:** Chromium helps enhance the effects of insulin, which may help reduce blood sugar levels and improve ovulation in women with PCOS.
- **Dosage:** 200–1,000 mcg per day is typical, but it's best to start low and increase as needed.

*8. Cinnamon*

- **Purpose:** Cinnamon has been shown to improve insulin sensitivity and regulate blood sugar.
- **How it Works:** Cinnamon slows glucose absorption in the bloodstream, which can help with insulin sensitivity and hormone regulation in PCOS.
- **Dosage:** Around 1-2 grams per day in supplement form or as a spice in meals.

*9. Berberine*

- **Purpose:** Berberine helps with insulin sensitivity, weight loss, and lowering androgen levels.
- **How it Works:** Berberine has similar effects to metformin (a common medication for PCOS), helping regulate blood sugar and insulin resistance. It also has anti-inflammatory properties.
- **Dosage:** 500 mg, two to three times per day, but it's essential to consult a healthcare provider before starting.

## HERBAL REMEDIES FOR PCOS

Several herbs are known for their hormone-balancing effects and can help with menstrual irregularity and symptoms of PCOS.

- **Vitex (Chasteberry):** Helps balance progesterone and estrogen levels, which may support menstrual regularity.
- **Spearmint Tea:** Known for its anti-androgen properties, spearmint tea

can help reduce testosterone levels and symptoms like hirsutism.

- **Licorice Root**: May help regulate estrogen levels and reduce androgen production, which can improve symptoms of PCOS.
- **White Peony and Licorice Root Combination:** This traditional herbal combination is used to support hormone balance, reduce testosterone, and improve fertility in women with PCOS.

# STEP 7: MENTAL HEALTH AND EMOTIONAL RESILIENCE

Living with PCOS can be challenging, both physically and emotionally. The symptoms, treatments, and ongoing health management that come with PCOS can often impact mental health, making resilience an essential component of navigating this condition. Here's how PCOS affects mental well-being and how resilience can help in managing these challenges:

### *1. Recognizing the Emotional Impact of PCOS*

PCOS is often accompanied by symptoms like weight gain, acne, hirsutism (excess hair growth), and fertility struggles. These physical manifestations can have a significant emotional impact, leading to feelings of frustration, embarrassment, and even shame. Many women with PCOS report feelings of isolation due to the lack of awareness about the condition. This can lead to mood swings, anxiety, and, in some cases, depression.

### *2. Building Self-Compassion and Self-Acceptance*

The visible symptoms of PCOS, such as weight gain and acne, can impact self-esteem and body image. Society often places immense pressure on women to look a certain way, which can exacerbate feelings of inadequacy for women with PCOS. Cultivating self-compassion—treating yourself with kindness and understanding rather than self-criticism—is key.

### *3. Developing a Healthy Relationship with Food and Exercise*

PCOS is commonly associated with insulin resistance, making it important to follow a balanced diet and maintain an active lifestyle. However, the need to "manage" weight and symptoms through diet and exercise can sometimes lead to a strained relationship with food or exercise, especially if results aren't immediately visible. This can create a cycle of frustration, stress, and self-criticism.

***4. Managing Stress and Reducing Anxiety***

PCOS can affect cortisol levels, increasing stress responses in the body. Additionally, managing PCOS symptoms and treatment can be overwhelming, leading to heightened anxiety. Stress itself can worsen PCOS symptoms, creating a vicious cycle that can feel challenging to break. Some stress management techniques are:

- **Yoga and Meditation:** Practicing yoga or meditation regularly helps reduce cortisol levels and may improve insulin sensitivity.
- **Mindfulness Techniques:** Practicing mindfulness or guided breathing can help with stress management.
- **Acupuncture:** Acupuncture has been shown to support hormone balance, reduce stress, and improve blood flow, which may help women with PCOS.

- **Consistent Sleep Schedule:** Going to bed and waking up at the same time each day.
- **Limiting Screen Time:** Reducing exposure to screens before bed can help improve sleep quality.
- **Creating a Relaxing Bedtime Routine:** Reading, gentle stretching, or meditation can support better sleep.

***5. Understanding the Impact of Hormones on Mood***

The hormonal imbalances of PCOS, including fluctuations in estrogen, progesterone, and androgens, can directly impact mood, leading to increased irritability, mood swings, and difficulty regulating emotions. These mood changes are not "all in your head"—they're real physiological reactions to hormone fluctuations.

***6. Seeking Professional Help***

Many women with PCOS may benefit from professional mental health support, such as counseling or therapy. Speaking with a mental health professional who understands chronic conditions like PCOS can provide valuable coping strategies, emotional support, and tools for managing stress and self-esteem challenges related to PCOS.

### *7. Embracing a Long-Term, Patient Approach*

Living with PCOS requires a long-term approach to symptom management and self-care. While lifestyle changes, medications, and treatments can all be beneficial, PCOS is a chronic condition that may require ongoing adjustments and patience. The journey with PCOS is often one of trial and error, which can be emotionally exhausting.

### *8. Focusing on Personal Growth and Strength*

PCOS is a challenging condition, but overcoming these challenges can build mental and emotional strength. Each obstacle faced and each self-care habit cultivated contributes to personal growth and resilience.

Building resilience while managing PCOS is a journey that involves both self-care and self-compassion. By focusing on emotional well-being, recognizing achievements, and finding a support network, you can empower yourself to face the challenges of PCOS with strength and positivity. Remember, resilience is about adapting, growing, and ultimately thriving, even in the face of PCOS!

# From One PCOS Warrior To Another

Thank you so much for taking the time to explore my first volume: PCOS Roadmap of 'Empowered Path to Pregnancy'. I hope that through these pages, you've found practical guidance, encouragement, and a sense of community on your journey with PCOS. Navigating the challenges of PCOS, especially when it comes to conception, can be overwhelming and lonely. But remember, you are not alone, and there are ways forward.

I wrote this guide not just to provide answers, but to offer hope and empowerment—because I truly believe in the power of knowledge, persistence, and self-care in achieving your dreams. Whether you're just starting to explore your options, or you've been working towards this goal for some time, trust in your body and your resilience.

*Be sure to look out for my next guide, coming soon!* I'll be diving even deeper into this journey, sharing all my go-to resources, tips, and the personal tools that helped me along the way. Thank you for allowing me to be a part of your journey. You have the strength and tools within you to take on this path, and I'm cheering for you every step of the way! Wishing you all the best as you move forward with hope and empowerment! YOU GOT THIS!

All the best,
Kelly

# ABOUT THE AUTHOR

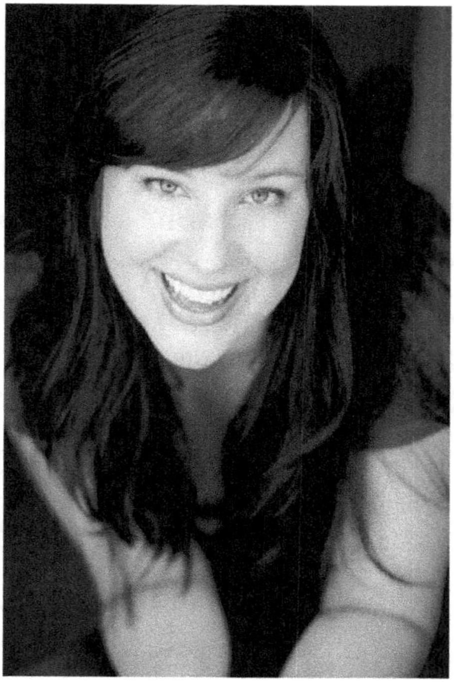

### How I Beat the Odds: My PCOS Journey to Motherhood

I was diagnosed with PCOS at 16 years old — a condition that, in the mid-90s, was largely overlooked and often misunderstood, even by many healthcare providers. At the time, all I knew was that PCOS was the cause of my irregular periods. It took years to connect all the other 'lovely' side effects—weight gain, acne, hair loss, Hirsutism (hair growth on face and body) to name a few.

Over the years, in an attempt to regulate my cycles, I was prescribed a rainbow of birth control pills but not one of them came without unbearable side effects. Frustrated, I decided to take myself off them and vowed to find a better way forward for my body. The journey was far from easy. I endured years of hormone imbalances and even had two colposcopies due to abnormal pap smears. For years, motherhood seemed like an elusive dream. But I didn't give up!

Through a blend of research, Western & Eastern medicine, lifestyle changes, and persistence, I finally balanced my hormones and regained regular cycles. At 39, I conceived naturally and welcomed a healthy baby at 40! In this guide, I'm thrilled to share the foundational steps to help you better understand and navigate PCOS. My hope is that this guide brings you clarity, encouragement, and a sense of empowerment to choose YOUR own path forward. Honestly, I wish I'd had a single, go-to guide like this to reference when I was working to conceive! If you find it helpful, stay tuned for my next guide, where I'll dive even deeper and share all my personal resources and go-to tools!

www.ingramcontent.com/pod-product-compliance
Lightning Source LLC
LaVergne TN
LVHW022313200926
848481LV00004B/1324